Primordial Nautilus Training: Expanding the Variable Method

By Steven Helmicki

ISBN: 978-0-557-28798-7

This is employment of Russian Shot put variable methodology to the use of first and second generation Nautilus Cam machines. Light to heavy alternating back and forth through exercise complexes. What better match for machines can be found than the original nautilus that Arthur Jones artfully left us utilizing a variable cam. Please pay close attention to changing lifting, holding and lowering counts. This is best achieved with a trainer or partner to rapidly change resistances and time the fatigued trainee to keep him or her within strict rest/hydration periods. Hydration is expected between each exercise and is to be conducted as rapidly as possible.

Record all workouts in the Primordial Strength System Training Log.

Train to Win. Period™

Workout U: perform the following movements in nautilus recommended protocol raise the weight on 2 count hold for one count lower on four count. Perform to momentary muscular failure. Between 12-18 repetitions.

Hip-Back

Leg extension

Leg press

Leg curl

Pullover

Pulldown

Decline press

Overhead press

Biceps

Triceps

Workout L- perform the following movements in nautilus recommended protocol raise the weight on 2 count hold for one count lower on four count. Perform to momentary muscular failure. Between 12-18 repetitions.

Ab-ductor and ad-ductor

Multi exercise squat

Multi-exercise stiff leg deadlift

Multi-exercise pull-ups

Multi-exercise chins

Multi exercise triceps extension with rope

Multi-exercise calf raises

Workout T- perform the following movements in nautilus recommended protocol raise the weight on 2 count hold for one count lower on four count. Perform to momentary muscular failure. Between 12-18 repetitions.

Leg press

Lateral raise

Arm cross

Rowing Torso

Shoulder/neck

4 way neck

Multi-exercise curl

Multi-exercise dip

Multi-exercise wrist curls

Workout I-select 50% of weight used in prior workout. Perform two reps and alternate back to 100% of weight used in prior workout. Alternate between weights in a light to heavy manner repeating it 5 times non-stop. Use the 2-1-4 count original nautilus methodology. Perform the entire workout in this manner.

Hip-Back

Leg extension

Leg press

Leg curl

Pullover

Pulldown

Decline press

Overhead press

Biceps

Triceps

Workout M- select 50% of weight used in prior workout. Perform two reps and alternate back to 100% of weight used in prior workout. Alternate between weights in a light to heavy manner repeating it 5 times non-stop. Use the 2-1-4 count original nautilus methodology. Perform the entire workout in this manner.

Ab-ductor and ad-ductor

Multi exercise squat

Multi-exercise stiff leg deadlift

Multi-exercise pull-ups

Multi-exercise chins

Multi exercise triceps extension with rope

Multi-exercise calf raises

Workout A- select 50% of weight used in prior workout. Perform two reps and alternate back to 100% of weight used in prior workout. Alternate between weights in a light to heavy manner repeating it 5 times non-stop. Use the 2-1-4 count original nautilus methodology. Perform the entire workout in this manner.

Leg press

Lateral raise

Arm cross

Rowing Torso

Shoulder/neck

4 way neck

Multi-exercise curl

Multi-exercise dip

Multi-exercise wrist curls

Workout T- Select a weight of 1/3 of the heaviest weight and perform 1 rep immediately followed by 2/3 of the heaviest weight and perform 1 rep followed by 100% of the heaviest weight x 1 alternating weights light to heavy repeating 7 times non-stop. Use the 2-1-4 count original nautilus methodology. Perform the entire workout in this manner.

Hip-Back

Leg extension

Leg press

Leg curl

Pullover

Pulldown

Decline press

Overhead press

Biceps

Triceps

Workout E- Select a weight of 1/3 of the heaviest weight and perform 1 rep immediately followed by 2/3 of the heaviest weight and perform 1 rep followed by 100% of the heaviest weight x 1 alternating weights light to heavy repeating 7 times non-stop. Use the 2-1-4 count original nautilus methodology. Perform the entire workout in this manner.

Ab-ductor and ad-ductor

Multi exercise squat

Multi-exercise stiff leg deadlift

Multi-exercise pull-ups

Multi-exercise chins

Multi exercise triceps extension with rope

Multi-exercise calf raises

Workout C- Select a weight of 1/3 of the heaviest weight and perform 1 rep immediately followed by 2/3 of the heaviest weight and perform 1 rep followed by 100% of the heaviest weight x 1 alternating weights light to heavy repeating 7 times non-stop. Use the 2-1-4 count original nautilus methodology. Perform the entire workout in this manner.

Leg press

Lateral raise

Arm cross

Rowing Torso

Shoulder/neck

4 way neck

Multi-exercise curl

Multi-exercise dip

Multi-exercise wrist curls

Workout L-Flush 1 plate on every machine and complete 100 reps. Use the 2-1-4 count original nautilus methodology. Perform the entire workout in this manner.

Hip-Back

Leg extension

Leg press

Leg curl

Pullover

Pulldown

Decline press

Overhead press

Biceps

Triceps

Workout U- Flush 1 plate on every machine and complete 100 reps. Use the 2-1-4 count original nautilus methodology. Perform the entire workout in this manner.

Ab-ductor and ad-ductor

Multi exercise squat

Multi-exercise stiff leg deadlift

Multi-exercise pull-ups

Multi-exercise chins

Multi exercise triceps extension with rope

Multi-exercise calf raises

Workout B- Flush 1 plate on every machine and complete 100 reps. Use the 2-1-4 count original nautilus methodology. Perform the entire workout in this manner.

Leg press

Lateral raise

Arm cross

Rowing Torso

Shoulder/neck

4 way neck

Multi-exercise curl

Multi-exercise dip

Multi-exercise wrist curls

Ultimate Club Introduction Complete.

Ultimate Primordial Nautilus Workout A- raise the weight on a 2 count, hold for 1 count and lower on a 2 count. Complete 2 reps on every 2 plate increment up to 100% of the weight used in Workout U. example: if 12 plates were used on the hip and back select 2 plates and perform 2 reps then with 4 plates then 2 reps with 6 plates then 2 reps with 8 plates then two reps with 10 plates and two reps with 12 plates. Repeat the complex three times.

Hip-Back

Leg extension

Leg press

Leg curl

Pullover

Pulldown

Decline press

Overhead press

Biceps

Triceps

Ultimate Primordial Nautilus Workout B- raise the weight on a 2 count, hold for 1 count and lower on a 2 count. Complete 2 reps on every 2 plate increment up to 100% of the weight used in Workout U. example: if 12 plates were used on the hip and back select 2 plates and perform 2 reps then with 4 plates then 2 reps with 6 plates then 2 reps with 8 plates then two reps with 10 plates and two reps with 12 plates. Repeat the complex three times.

Ab-ductor and ad-ductor

Multi exercise squat

Multi-exercise stiff leg deadlift

Multi-exercise pull-ups

Multi-exercise chins

Multi exercise triceps extension with rope

Multi-exercise calf raises

Ultimate Primordial Nautilus Workout C-raise the weight on a 2 count, hold for 1 count and lower on a 2 count. Complete 2 reps on every 2 plate increment up to 100% of the weight used in Workout U. example: if 12 plates were used on the hip and back select 2 plates and perform 2 reps then with 4 plates then 2 reps with 6 plates then 2 reps with 8 plates then two reps with 10 plates and two reps with 12 plates. Repeat the complex three times

Leg press

Lateral raise

Arm cross

Rowing Torso

Shoulder/neck

4 way neck

Multi-exercise curl

Multi-exercise dip

Multi-exercise wrist curls

Re-engineering the entire process. Start with higher weights for Workout U and re-calculate the entire programming based on your new numbers.

Workout U: perform the following movements in nautilus recommended protocol raise the weight on 2 count hold for one count lower on four count. Perform to momentary muscular failure. Between 12-18 repetitions.

Hip-Back

Leg extension

Leg press

Leg curl

Pullover

Pulldown

Decline press

Overhead press

Biceps

Triceps

Workout L- perform the following movements in nautilus recommended protocol raise the weight on 2 count hold for one count lower on four count. Perform to momentary muscular failure. Between 12-18 repetitions.

Ab-ductor and ad-ductor

Multi exercise squat

Multi-exercise stiff leg deadlift

Multi-exercise pull-ups

Multi-exercise chins

Multi exercise triceps extension with rope

Multi-exercise calf raises

Workout T- perform the following movements in nautilus recommended protocol raise the weight on 2 count hold for one count lower on four count. Perform to momentary muscular failure. Between 12-18 repetitions.

Leg press

Lateral raise

Arm cross

Rowing Torso

Shoulder/neck

4 way neck

Multi-exercise curl

Multi-exercise dip

Multi-exercise wrist curls

Workout I-select 50% of weight used in prior workout. Perform two reps and alternate back to 100% of weight used in prior workout. Alternate between weights in a light to heavy manner repeating it 5 times non-stop. Use the 2-1-4 count original nautilus methodology. Perform the entire workout in this manner.

Hip-Back

Leg extension

Leg press

Leg curl

Pullover

Pulldown

Decline press

Overhead press

Biceps

Triceps

Workout M- select 50% of weight used in prior workout. Perform two reps and alternate back to 100% of weight used in prior workout. Alternate between weights in a light to heavy manner repeating it 5 times non-stop. Use the 2-1-4 count original nautilus methodology. Perform the entire workout in this manner.

Ab-ductor and ad-ductor

Multi exercise squat

Multi-exercise stiff leg deadlift

Multi-exercise pull-ups

Multi-exercise chins

Multi exercise triceps extension with rope

Multi-exercise calf raises

Workout A- select 50% of weight used in prior workout. Perform two reps and alternate back to 100% of weight used in prior workout. Alternate between weights in a light to heavy manner repeating it 5 times non-stop. Use the 2-1-4 count original nautilus methodology. Perform the entire workout in this manner.

Leg press

Lateral raise

Arm cross

Rowing Torso

Shoulder/neck

4 way neck

Multi-exercise curl

Multi-exercise dip

Multi-exercise wrist curls

Workout T- Select a weight of 1/3 of the heaviest weight and perform 1 rep immediately followed by 2/3 of the heaviest weight and perform 1 rep followed by 100% of the heaviest weight x 1 alternating weights light to heavy repeating 7 times non-stop. Use the 2-1-4 count original nautilus methodology. Perform the entire workout in this manner.

Hip-Back

Leg extension

Leg press

Leg curl

Pullover

Pulldown

Decline press

Overhead press

Biceps

Triceps

Workout E- Select a weight of 1/3 of the heaviest weight and perform 1 rep immediately followed by 2/3 of the heaviest weight and perform 1 rep followed by 100% of the heaviest weight x 1 alternating weights light to heavy repeating 7 times non-stop. Use the 2-1-4 count original nautilus methodology. Perform the entire workout in this manner.

Ab-ductor and ad-ductor

Multi exercise squat

Multi-exercise stiff leg deadlift

Multi-exercise pull-ups

Multi-exercise chins

Multi exercise triceps extension with rope

Multi-exercise calf raises

Workout C- Select a weight of 1/3 of the heaviest weight and perform 1 rep immediately followed by 2/3 of the heaviest weight and perform 1 rep followed by 100% of the heaviest weight x 1 alternating weights light to heavy repeating 7 times non-stop. Use the 2-1-4 count original nautilus methodology. Perform the entire workout in this manner.

Leg press

Lateral raise

Arm cross

Rowing Torso

Shoulder/neck

4 way neck

Multi-exercise curl

Multi-exercise dip

Multi-exercise wrist curls

Workout L-Flush 1 plate on every machine and complete 100 reps. Use the 2-1-4 count original nautilus methodology. Perform the entire workout in this manner.

Hip-Back

Leg extension

Leg press

Leg curl

Pullover

Pulldown

Decline press

Overhead press

Biceps

Triceps

Workout U- Flush 1 plate on every machine and complete 100 reps. Use the 2-1-4 count original nautilus methodology. Perform the entire workout in this manner.

Ab-ductor and ad-ductor

Multi exercise squat

Multi-exercise stiff leg deadlift

Multi-exercise pull-ups

Multi-exercise chins

Multi exercise triceps extension with rope

Multi-exercise calf raises

Workout B- Flush 1 plate on every machine and complete 100 reps. Use the 2-1-4 count original nautilus methodology. Perform the entire workout in this manner.

Leg press

Lateral raise

Arm cross

Rowing Torso

Shoulder/neck

4 way neck

Multi-exercise curl

Multi-exercise dip

Multi-exercise wrist curls

Ultimate Club Membership Gained.

Ultimate Primordial Nautilus Workout A- raise the weight on a 2 count, hold for 1 count and lower on a 2 count. Complete 2 reps on every 2 plate increment up to 100% of the weight used in Workout U. example: if 12 plates were used on the hip and back select 2 plates and perform 2 reps then with 4 plates then 2 reps with 6 plates then 2 reps with 8 plates then two reps with 10 plates and two reps with 12 plates. Repeat the complex three times.

Hip-Back

Leg extension

Leg press

Leg curl

Pullover

Pulldown

Decline press

Overhead press

Biceps

Triceps

Ultimate Primordial Nautilus Workout B- raise the weight on a 2 count, hold for 1 count and lower on a 2 count. Complete 2 reps on every 2 plate increment up to 100% of the weight used in Workout U. example: if 12 plates were used on the hip and back select 2 plates and perform 2 reps then with 4 plates then 2 reps with 6 plates then 2 reps with 8 plates then two reps with 10 plates and two reps with 12 plates. Repeat the complex three times.

Ab-ductor and ad-ductor

Multi exercise squat

Multi-exercise stiff leg deadlift

Multi-exercise pull-ups

Multi-exercise chins

Multi exercise triceps extension with rope

Multi-exercise calf raises

Ultimate Primordial Nautilus Workout C-raise the weight on a 2 count, hold for 1 count and lower on a 2 count. Complete 2 reps on every 2 plate increment up to 100% of the weight used in Workout U. example: if 12 plates were used on the hip and back select 2 plates and perform 2 reps then with 4 plates then 2 reps with 6 plates then 2 reps with 8 plates then two reps with 10 plates and two reps with 12 plates. Repeat the complex three times

Leg press

Lateral raise

Arm cross

Rowing Torso

Shoulder/neck

4 way neck

Multi-exercise curl

Multi-exercise dip

Multi-exercise wrist curls